Contents

Introduction:

Welcome to **"The Ultimate Guide for Healthy Living & Eating Habits."** In a world brimming with information, this concise yet comprehensive E-book is your roadmap to a transformed lifestyle. Discover the symbiotic relationship between your well-being and daily choices, as we delve into the realms of nutrition, exercise, mental clarity, and more. Unearth the power of mindful eating, sustainable habits, and holistic self-care. Whether you're a seasoned wellness enthusiast or taking your first steps towards a healthier you, this guide will equip you with practical insights and actionable steps to embrace vitality, one habit at a time. Your journey to lasting wellness begins here.

The importance of healthy living and eating habits:

Embracing healthy living and adopting nourishing eating habits is paramount for overall well-being. Our modern lifestyle is marked by hectic schedules, sedentary routines, and processed foods, leading to a host of health challenges. In this context, the significance of healthy living cannot be overstated.

Healthy living encompasses physical, mental, and emotional health, fostering a balanced and thriving existence. A nutritious diet fuels our bodies with essential nutrients, supporting bodily functions and bolstering our immune systems. It plays a pivotal role in preventing chronic diseases such as obesity, diabetes, and heart ailments. Moreover, proper nutrition directly influences cognitive function and emotional stability, affecting our productivity, mood, and ability to manage stress.

Coupled with a balanced diet, regular exercise amplifies the benefits of healthy living. It enhances cardiovascular health, strengthens muscles and bones, and improves mental clarity. Engaging in physical activity releases endorphins, the "feel-good" hormones, which contribute to reduced anxiety and enhanced mental well-being.

Healthy living isn't a short-term goal; it's a sustainable lifestyle that engenders longevity and vitality. By prioritizing wholesome foods, engaging in regular exercise, nurturing quality sleep, and managing stress effectively, we pave the way for a higher quality of life. In this holistic approach to health, we empower ourselves to seize each day with Vigor and embrace a future of wellness. The choices we make today resonate in our tomorrows, making the cultivation of healthy living and eating habits a vital investment in ourselves and our future.

How this guide will help transform your lifestyle:

This guide is your catalyst for transformative change. By distilling essential principles of healthy living and eating habits, it empowers you to revitalize your lifestyle. Through practical advice and proven strategies, you'll attain a deeper understanding of nutrition, exercise, and holistic well-being. Unlock the potential to make informed choices, establish sustainable routines, and foster a harmonious mind-body connection. As you embark on this journey, you'll witness the gradual evolution of your habits, resulting in increased energy, improved resilience, and a renewed zest for life. This guide is your steadfast companion, propelling you toward a truly transformative and lasting lifestyle change.

Chapter 1: Understanding Healthy Living:

- Defining healthy living and its components
- The connection between physical, mental, and emotional well-being
- Benefits of adopting a healthy lifestyle

In the journey towards holistic well-being, "Understanding Healthy Living" serves as the foundational chapter, unveiling the core principles that shape a vibrant and balanced lifestyle.

Defining Healthy Living and Its Components:

Healthy living transcends mere absence of illness; it encapsulates a state of complete physical, mental, and emotional well-being. It encompasses a harmonious synergy between these dimensions. Physical health involves maintaining a well-functioning body through proper nutrition, regular exercise, and adequate rest. Mental health pertains to cognitive well-being, encompassing clarity of thought, emotional resilience, and effective stress management. Emotional health is rooted in acknowledging and nurturing our feelings, fostering healthy relationships, and developing coping mechanisms.

The Connection Between Physical, Mental, and Emotional Well-being:

The inseparable connection between these facets cannot be overstated. Physical exercise, for instance, not only enhances cardiovascular health but also releases endorphins, elevating mood and reducing stress. A balanced diet rich in essential nutrients not only fuels our bodies but also supports cognitive function and emotional stability. Moreover, the mind-body connection highlights that mental and emotional states impact physical health; chronic stress can manifest as physical ailments.

Benefits of Adopting a Healthy Lifestyle:

Embarking on a journey towards healthy living brings forth an array of benefits. Enhanced physical vitality translates to increased energy, reduced risk of chronic diseases, and improved longevity. Mental clarity and emotional resilience empower us to navigate life's challenges with grace and poise. By cultivating healthy habits, we gain a sense of empowerment and control over our well-being, fostering a positive self-image and bolstering confidence.

In conclusion, "Understanding Healthy Living" lays the groundwork for a transformative journey. By acknowledging the interplay between physical, mental, and emotional dimensions, we embrace a holistic approach that enables us to harness the full spectrum of our potential. The benefits extend far beyond individual well-being, radiating positively into all aspects of our lives. This chapter sets the tone for the subsequent exploration of practical strategies, making the pursuit of a balanced and fulfilling life an achievable reality.

Chapter 2: Building a Strong Foundation:

- Setting clear goals for your health journey
- Creating a personalized plan for success
- Overcoming obstacles and staying motivated

In the pursuit of a healthier lifestyle, "Building a Strong Foundation" serves as a pivotal chapter that equips you with the tools and insights to lay the groundwork for lasting change.

Setting Clear Goals for Your Health Journey:

Goal setting is the compass that guides your health journey. By defining specific, measurable, achievable, relevant, and time-bound (SMART) goals, you establish a clear path towards your desired outcomes. Whether your goals involve weight loss, increased fitness, or improved mental clarity, clarity in goal-setting enhances focus and commitment. Clearly defined goals provide direction and a sense of purpose, acting as a source of motivation during challenging times.

Creating a Personalized Plan for Success:

A one-size-fits-all approach doesn't apply to healthy living. Crafting a personalized plan tailored to your individual preferences, needs, and circumstances is essential. Consider your current habits, preferences, dietary requirements, and any health concerns. This plan should encompass a balanced diet, regular exercise, sufficient sleep, and strategies for managing stress. A well-structured plan increases the likelihood of sustainable success by aligning with your unique lifestyle.

Overcoming Obstacles and Staying Motivated:

Obstacles are inevitable, but they needn't derail your progress. Identifying potential challenges such as time constraints, cravings, or a busy schedule empowers you to devise strategies to overcome them.

Seek support from friends, family, or professionals if needed. Staying motivated requires cultivating a positive mindset. Regularly revisit your goals, track your progress, and celebrate small victories. Incorporate motivational practices like visualization, positive affirmations, and mindfulness to keep your determination high.

By developing a solid foundation through goal-setting, personalized planning, and motivation strategies, you set yourself up for success. Remember that building healthy habits is a gradual process, and setbacks are natural. Adaptability and resilience are key as you navigate challenges and refine your approach. This chapter empowers you to take charge of your health journey, transforming aspirations into tangible results. As you construct this strong foundation, you're setting the stage for sustainable, positive change that will shape your life for years to come.

Chapter 3: Nourishing Your Body:

- The basics of nutrition: macronutrients and micronutrients
- Portion control and mindful eating
- Designing a balanced and varied diet

In the intricate tapestry of healthy living, the thread of nutrition weaves a foundation of vitality and well-being. This chapter delves into the art and science of nourishing your body, exploring the fundamental components that fuel your daily life.

The Basics of Nutrition: Macronutrients and Micronutrients

Nutrition is the cornerstone of a thriving existence, and understanding its building blocks is essential. Macronutrients—carbohydrates, proteins, and fats—provide the energy required for bodily functions. Carbohydrates are the primary energy source, while proteins facilitate growth and repair, and fats support cellular integrity and hormone production. Micronutrients—vitamins and minerals—play a pivotal role in various physiological processes, bolstering immunity, bone health, and more.

Portion Control and Mindful Eating

Portion control is a key strategy in maintaining a balanced diet. Overeating, even with nutritious foods, can lead to weight gain. Mindful eating cultivates a conscious connection with your food. Engage your senses, savor each bite, and eat slowly to give your body time to signal when it's full. Avoid distractions during meals, such as screens or work, allowing you to be attuned to your body's hunger and satiety cues.

Designing a Balanced and Varied Diet

A balanced diet draws from a spectrum of foods, ensuring that your body receives a wide array of nutrients. Prioritize whole foods— fruits, vegetables, whole grains, lean proteins, and healthy fats. Aim for a colorful plate, as different colors signify different nutrients. Incorporate foods rich in fiber to support digestion and satiety. Experiment with different cuisines and cooking methods to keep your meals exciting and diverse.

Creating a Nutrient-Rich Plate: The Healthy Plate Model

A useful framework for meal planning is the Healthy Plate Model. Imagine your plate divided into sections: half for vegetables and fruits, a quarter for lean proteins, and a quarter for whole grains or starchy vegetables. Add a source of healthy fat, like nuts or olive oil, to complete the picture. This model ensures a balanced intake of macronutrients and micronutrients, promoting overall well-being.

Navigating Dietary Preferences and Restrictions

Individual dietary preferences and restrictions vary, but the principles of nutrition remain constant. Vegetarians and vegans can obtain essential nutrients through plant-based sources such as legumes, nuts, and fortified foods. Those with gluten intolerance or allergies should explore gluten-free grains like quinoa, rice, and oats. If you have specific health conditions, consult a healthcare professional or registered dietitian to tailor your diet accordingly.

The Power of Hydration: Water as a Vital Nutrient

Water is often overlooked but is critical for overall health. It aids in digestion, nutrient transport, temperature regulation, and more. Aim to drink water throughout the day, and pay attention to your body's signals for thirst. Herbal teas and infused water can add variety and flavor to your hydration routine.

The Role of Dietary Supplements

While a well-rounded diet should be your primary source of nutrients, certain situations may warrant supplementation. Vitamin D, omega-3 fatty acids, and specific vitamins or minerals may be recommended by healthcare professionals. However, supplements should not replace a balanced diet and should be taken under supervision.

Cultivating a Healthy Relationship with Food

Nourishing your body involves not just the physical aspect but also the psychological and emotional elements of your relationship with food. Avoid extreme diets, as they are often unsustainable and can lead to a cycle of restriction and overindulgence. Practice self-compassion and strive for balance rather than perfection. Seek joy in eating by savouring Flavors and embracing occasional indulgences without guilt.

Meal Planning and Preparation

Efficient meal planning and preparation streamline your journey towards better nutrition. Set aside time to plan meals for the week, create shopping lists, and prepare ingredients in advance. Batch cooking can save time on busy days, ensuring that you have nutritious options readily available.

In the intricate dance of nourishing your body, the choreography lies in understanding the essentials of nutrition, practicing mindful eating, and curating a balanced diet that celebrates both health and pleasure. This chapter illuminates the path to making informed choices, forging a relationship with food that not only sustains your physical self but enriches your entire well-being. As you embark on this voyage, remember that nutrition is not a destination but a continuous journey of learning, adapting, and growing towards a vibrant life.

Chapter 4: Supercharging Your Diet with Whole Foods:

- Exploring the benefits of whole, unprocessed foods
- Incorporating fruits and vegetables for optimal health
- Grains, legumes, and lean protein sources: building blocks of a nutritious diet.

In a world brimming with culinary choices, the path to optimal health often begins with one simple principle: embracing whole, unprocessed foods. This chapter takes you on a journey through the vibrant realm of whole foods, revealing their undeniable impact on nourishment, vitality, and overall well-being.

Exploring the Benefits of Whole, Unprocessed Foods

Whole foods are nature's gift, brimming with essential nutrients and devoid of additives, preservatives, and artificial flavourings. The journey from farm to table preserves the integrity of these foods, ensuring that they retain their natural goodness. The benefits are manifold: improved nutrient absorption, sustained energy levels, enhanced digestion, and a reduced risk of chronic diseases.

Incorporating Fruits and Vegetables for Optimal Health

Fruits and vegetables stand as the cornerstone of a nutrient-rich diet. Bursting with vitamins, minerals, fibre, and antioxidants, they fortify your body's defence against oxidative stress and inflammation. Their vibrant colours reflect their diverse nutrient profiles. Aim for a rainbow on your plate, embracing the spectrum of colors from deep greens to vivid reds and oranges. Incorporating these plant-based powerhouses fuels your body with essential vitamins and minerals while supporting a healthy immune system.

Grains, Legumes, and Lean Protein Sources: Building Blocks of a Nutritious Diet

Whole grains and legumes provide sustained energy and are rich sources of dietary fiber, essential for digestive health. Quinoa, brown rice, oats, and whole wheat are among the grains that offer a spectrum of nutrients. Legumes such as beans, lentils, and chickpeas provide plant-based proteins, fiber, and a medley of vitamins and minerals.

Lean protein sources play a crucial role in muscle repair and overall well-being. Incorporate lean cuts of poultry, fish, tofu, tempeh, and low-fat dairy to provide essential amino acids while minimizing saturated fats. These sources of lean protein contribute to satiety, helping you maintain a balanced diet and manage weight effectively.

Navigating the World of Healthy Fats

Healthy fats are integral to bodily functions and should not be avoided. Sources such as avocados, nuts, seeds, and olive oil provide heart-healthy monounsaturated and polyunsaturated fats. These fats support brain health, hormone production, and absorption of fat-soluble vitamins.

Mindful Eating: A Catalyst for Wholesome Nourishment

Incorporating whole foods extends beyond ingredients; it embraces a mindful approach to eating. Mindful eating encourages you to savor each bite, fostering an intimate connection with your food and recognizing cues of hunger and fullness. By slowing down and relishing the flavors and textures, you enhance digestion and prevent overeating.

Practical Tips for Incorporating Whole Foods

- Plan your meals around whole ingredients.
- Shop the perimeter of grocery stores where fresh produce is often located.
- Prioritize seasonal and local produce for enhanced nutrient density.
- Experiment with new recipes to diversify your diet.
- Limit highly processed foods that tend to be high in added sugars, sodium, and unhealthy fats.

The Art of Food Preparation: From Garden to Plate

Growing your own fruits, vegetables, and herbs fosters a deep connection with your food. Even a small garden or potted herbs can offer an array of fresh ingredients. Engaging in food preparation, from chopping vegetables to crafting wholesome meals, becomes an act of nourishment and creativity.

Cultivating Culinary Creativity

Whole foods invite you to experiment with flavors, textures, and cooking methods. Roasting, steaming, sautéing, and blending are techniques that preserve the nutritional integrity of ingredients. Expand your culinary horizons by trying new ingredients and exploring various cuisines that celebrate the goodness of whole foods.

As you embark on this journey of supercharging your diet with whole foods, remember that each plate holds the potential to nourish not only your body but also your soul. By embracing the simplicity and abundance of nature's bounty, you tap into a source of vitality that transcends calories and nutrients. Whole foods become not just sustenance, but a celebration of life, health, and the journey towards lasting well-being.

Chapter 5: Hydration and Its Impact:

- The importance of staying hydrated
- Choosing the right beverages for your health
- Tips for maintaining proper hydration throughout the day

Water, the elixir of life, forms the foundation of vitality and well-being. In this chapter, we explore the crucial role of hydration in sustaining health, the art of making mindful beverage choices, and strategies for ensuring optimal hydration throughout your day.

The Importance of Staying Hydrated

Water is the essence of life, constituting a significant portion of our bodies and performing a myriad of essential functions. It regulates body temperature, aids digestion, facilitates nutrient transport, and supports cellular processes. Adequate hydration is fundamental for maintaining proper bodily functions, from cognition to circulation.

Understanding Your Body's Hydration Needs

Your body continually loses water through processes such as sweating, breathing, and urination. Therefore, replenishing this loss is crucial. Factors like age, physical activity, climate, and health conditions influence your hydration needs. Ignoring these needs can lead to dehydration, marked by symptoms such as fatigue, headaches, dizziness, and decreased cognitive function.

Choosing the Right Beverages for Your Health

While water remains the optimal choice for hydration, other beverages can also contribute to your fluid intake. Unsweetened herbal teas, infused water, and beverages with high water content foods like fruits and vegetables are beneficial alternatives. Beware of sugary drinks and excessive caffeine consumption, as they can disrupt your hydration balance. Alcoholic beverages can also lead to dehydration; it's essential to consume them in moderation and balance them with water.

Beyond Water: Nutrient-Rich Hydration

Some beverages not only hydrate but also offer additional health benefits. Freshly squeezed juices, smoothies, and coconut water can provide vitamins, minerals, and electrolytes. Herbal teas, like chamomile or peppermint, offer soothing properties. Green tea is celebrated for its antioxidants and potential metabolism-boosting effects. When incorporating these beverages, consider their nutritional content and consume them mindfully.

Tips for Maintaining Proper Hydration Throughout the Day

- **Carry a Water Bottle:** Having a reusable water bottle on hand encourages consistent sipping throughout the day.
- **Set Hydration Goals:** Aim for a certain volume of water intake based on your needs. Using cues like thirst, urine color, and body weight can help gauge hydration status.
- **Infuse Your Water:** Enhance the flavor of water with slices of citrus fruits, berries, cucumbers, or mint leaves.
- **Hydrate Before, During, and After Exercise:** Physical activity increases fluid loss through sweat. Hydrate before exercising, drink water during activity, and replenish post-workout.

- **Create Hydration Triggers:** Link hydration to routine activities like waking up, before meals, and during breaks.
- **Eat Hydrating Foods:** Foods with high water content, such as watermelon, cucumber, and lettuce, contribute to your overall hydration.
- **Limit Caffeine and Sugary Drinks:** These beverages can have a diuretic effect, leading to increased fluid loss.
- **Monitor Hydration During Hot Weather:** In warmer climates or during strenuous activities, increase fluid intake to compensate for higher sweat rates.

Cultivating Mindful Hydration Habits

Hydration extends beyond mere consumption; it embodies a mindful practice. Sip water intentionally, savoring each drop and acknowledging the essential role it plays in your well-being. As you become attuned to your body's signals, you empower yourself to meet its hydration needs with care and precision.

Hydration and the Mind-Body Connection

The relationship between hydration and mental clarity is profound. Dehydration can lead to cognitive decline, decreased concentration, and mood disturbances. Hydrating your body isn't just about quenching physical thirst; it's about nurturing your mental acuity and emotional equilibrium.

Conclusion: Embracing the Gift of Hydration

Hydration is a simple yet potent act of self-care. By prioritizing hydration, you gift your body with the essence of life, a foundation for vitality and health. The journey towards optimal hydration is one of mindfulness, intention, and reverence for your body's needs. With every sip, you not only quench your thirst but also reaffirm your commitment to a life of well-being and vitality.

Chapter 6: The Role of Exercise in Healthy Living:

- Different types of exercise and their benefits
- Creating a personalized workout routine

- Incorporating physical activity into your daily life

Movement is an intrinsic aspect of the human experience, contributing not only to physical health but also to mental and emotional well-being. This chapter delves into the multifaceted role of exercise in promoting a holistic sense of vitality, guiding you through various types of exercise, the creation of a personalized workout routine, and integrating physical activity seamlessly into your daily life.

Understanding Different Types of Exercise and Their Benefits

Exercise encompasses a diverse spectrum of activities, each offering unique benefits for your body and mind.

- **Cardiovascular (Aerobic) Exercise:** Activities like running, cycling, and swimming elevate your heart rate, improving cardiovascular health, endurance, and calorie burn.
- **Strength Training:** Lifting weights, resistance band exercises, and bodyweight workouts enhance muscle strength, metabolism, bone density, and overall functional capacity.
- **Flexibility and Mobility Exercises:** Yoga, Pilates, and stretching routines enhance flexibility, joint range of motion, and balance while reducing the risk of injury.
- **Mind-Body Practices:** Tai chi and qigong blend movement with mindfulness, promoting relaxation, stress reduction, and mind-body connection.
- **High-Intensity Interval Training (HIIT):** Alternating between high-intensity bursts and rest periods, HIIT improves cardiovascular fitness, burns calories, and can be time-efficient.

Creating a Personalized Workout Routine

Designing a workout routine that aligns with your goals, preferences, and fitness level is essential for consistency and progress.

- **Set Clear Goals:** Determine whether you aim to lose weight, build muscle, improve endurance, or enhance flexibility. Your goals will shape the structure of your routine.

- **Balance Variety and Consistency:** Include a mix of exercises to engage different muscle groups and prevent monotony. However, consistency is key; establish a routine you can commit to.
- **Frequency and Duration:** Aim for at least 150 minutes of moderate-intensity aerobic exercise or 75 minutes of vigorous-intensity exercise per week, along with two days of strength training.
- **Progressive Overload:** Gradually increase the intensity, duration, or weight of your exercises to challenge your body and foster improvement.
- **Rest and Recovery:** Integrate rest days into your routine to allow your muscles to recover and prevent burnout.

Incorporating Physical Activity into Your Daily Life

Movement need not be confined to formal workouts; integrating physical activity into your daily routine enhances overall well-being.

- **Active Commuting:** Walk or cycle to work if feasible or use public transportation for part of the journey.
- **Take Active Breaks:** Stand up, stretch, or take a brisk walk during breaks at work to counteract sedentary behaviour.
- **Stairs Instead of Elevators:** Opt for stairs whenever possible, promoting cardiovascular fitness and muscle engagement.
- **Leisure Activities:** Engage in hobbies that involve movement, such as dancing, gardening, or playing a sport.
- **Family Time:** Make physical activity a family affair by going for walks, bike rides, or participating in active games.
- **Mindful Movement:** Practice mindfulness through walking meditation, where each step is deliberate and focused.

The Mind-Body Connection: Exercise and Mental Well-being

Exercise goes beyond physical benefits; it profoundly impacts mental and emotional well-being.

Endorphin Release: Physical activity stimulates the release of endorphins, the "feel-good" hormones that alleviate stress, improve mood, and boost overall happiness.

Reduced Anxiety and Depression: Regular exercise is associated with a decreased risk of anxiety and depression, promoting mental resilience.

Enhanced Cognitive Function: Exercise improves cognitive function, memory, and focus by increasing blood flow to the brain.

Stress Reduction: Engaging in physical activity provides an outlet for stress and helps manage its effects on the body.

Overcoming Barriers and Cultivating a Positive Mindset

Numerous barriers, from time constraints to lack of motivation, can hinder your exercise routine. Overcoming these challenges requires cultivating a positive mindset.

Set Realistic Expectations: Avoid setting unrealistic goals; instead, focus on steady progress and gradual improvement.

Adapt and Be Flexible: Life is dynamic, and your routine should be adaptable. Modify your workouts based on changes in your schedule or physical condition.

Find Joy in Movement: Choose activities you enjoy, ensuring that exercise becomes a source of pleasure rather than a chore.

Accountability and Support: Seek accountability through workout partners, fitness classes, or fitness apps that track your progress.

Listen to Your Body: Rest when needed, and pay attention to signals of fatigue or pain to prevent injury.

Conclusion: The Ever-Evolving Journey of Movement

Exercise is not a destination but a journey, an ongoing exploration of your body's capabilities and the limitless potential within. It's a celebration of what your body can achieve, fostering vitality, strength, and resilience. By embracing a diverse array of physical activities, crafting a personalized routine, and weaving movement into the fabric of your daily life, you embark on a transformative path of holistic well-being. This chapter invites you to dance through life with vigor, honoring the symphony of movement that nourishes body, mind, and soul.

Chapter 7: Prioritizing Sleep and Rest:

- Understanding the importance of quality sleep
- Establishing a sleep-friendly environment
- Techniques for improving sleep and managing stress

In the relentless rhythm of modern life, sleep often takes a backseat to demanding schedules and constant connectivity. Yet, quality sleep and rest are pillars of well-being, essential for physical health, mental clarity, and emotional equilibrium. This chapter delves into the significance of sleep, unveils the art of creating a restful sleep environment, and equips you with techniques to optimize your sleep quality while effectively managing stress.

Understanding the Importance of Quality Sleep

Sleep is not merely a passive state of inactivity; it's a dynamic process that rejuvenates your body and mind. During sleep, essential processes unfold, including tissue repair, memory consolidation, and hormone regulation. Adequate sleep is linked to improved cognitive function, enhanced mood, strengthened immunity, and lowered risk of chronic diseases.

The Science of Sleep Cycles

Sleep occurs in cycles, consisting of rapid eye movement (REM) and non-REM stages. Each cycle is characterized by distinct physiological and brain activity patterns. Deep, restorative sleep primarily occurs during non-REM stages, while REM sleep is associated with vivid dreams and cognitive restoration. Aim for 7-9 hours of sleep per night to ensure you traverse these cycles for optimal rejuvenation.

Establishing a Sleep-Friendly Environment

Creating an environment conducive to sleep is essential for maximizing restfulness and sleep quality.

- **Darkness and Light:** Ensure your sleep environment is dark during bedtime to encourage melatonin production, a hormone that regulates sleep. In the morning, expose yourself to natural sunlight to synchronize your circadian rhythm.

- **Comfortable Bedding:** Invest in a comfortable mattress and pillows that support your body's needs, ensuring you wake up refreshed.
- **Temperature Control:** Maintain a comfortable room temperature, as both extremes can disrupt sleep.
- **Limit Noise:** Minimize disruptive sounds using earplugs, white noise machines, or calming music if needed.
- **Digital Detox:** Create a technology-free zone in your bedroom to limit exposure to screens, which emit blue light that interferes with melatonin production.

Techniques for Improving Sleep and Managing Stress

- **Establish a Consistent Sleep Schedule:** Go to bed and wake up at the same time every day, even on weekends. Consistency reinforces your body's internal clock.
- **Mindfulness and Relaxation Techniques:** Engage in relaxation techniques such as deep breathing, progressive muscle relaxation, or meditation to unwind before bed.
- **Limit Stimulants:** Reduce caffeine and alcohol intake close to bedtime, as they can disrupt sleep patterns.
- **Screen Time Reduction:** Diminish screen time at least an hour before sleep to minimize the impact of blue light on melatonin production.
- **Physical Activity:** Regular exercise promotes restful sleep, but avoid vigorous activity close to bedtime, as it may energize you.
- **Evening Rituals:** Create soothing rituals before sleep, such as reading, taking a warm bath, or practicing gentle stretches.
- **Nutrition:** Avoid heavy meals close to bedtime, as digestion can interfere with sleep. Opt for light, easily digestible snacks if needed.
- **Limit Naps:** While short naps can be refreshing, lengthy naps during the day may disrupt nighttime sleep.

The Connection Between Sleep and Stress Management

Stress and sleep are interconnected; poor sleep can exacerbate stress, while high stress levels can disrupt sleep. To foster a balanced relationship between the two:

- **Stress Management Techniques:** Incorporate stress-relief practices like yoga, meditation, journaling, or spending time in nature to create emotional equilibrium.
- **Prioritize Relaxation:** Designate time for relaxation before sleep to transition from a state of alertness to restfulness.
- **Address Worries:** If racing thoughts prevent sleep, jot down your concerns in a journal and remind yourself that you can address them tomorrow.

Sleep as a Pillar of Holistic Well-being

Prioritizing sleep is not indulgence; it's an investment in your well-being. In a world that glorifies productivity and busy schedules, embracing sleep as a vital pillar of holistic health empowers you to navigate life with clarity, resilience, and vitality. By creating a sleep-friendly environment and practicing stress management techniques, you reclaim your nights as a sanctuary for restoration and renewal. This chapter invites you to honor sleep as a cherished gift, a path to unlocking your full potential and embracing a life of optimal well-being.

Chapter 8: Mental and Emotional Well-being:

- The mind-body connection in health
- Strategies for managing stress and anxiety
- Practicing mindfulness and meditation

In the intricate dance of well-being, the harmony between the mind and body holds profound significance. This chapter illuminates the powerful interplay between mental and emotional health and physical well-being. It delves into strategies for effectively managing stress and anxiety, and it guides you through the transformative practices of mindfulness and meditation, offering tools to cultivate a state of equilibrium and vitality.

The Mind-Body Connection in Health

The intricate relationship between the mind and body is a cornerstone of holistic well-being. Thoughts, emotions, and physiological responses are interwoven, impacting each other in a delicate symphony. Positive emotions foster physical health, while chronic stress and negative emotions can manifest as physical ailments. Understanding this connection empowers you to embrace a holistic approach that nurtures both mental and physical vitality.

Strategies for Managing Stress and Anxiety

In the modern whirlwind of responsibilities, stress and anxiety can become unwelcome companions. Adopting effective strategies to manage these emotions is essential for maintaining equilibrium.

- **Identify Stressors:** Recognize the triggers of stress and anxiety in your life. By acknowledging their sources, you can devise targeted coping strategies.
- **Practice Time Management:** Organize your tasks and allocate time efficiently to reduce the pressure of looming deadlines.
- **Embrace Self-Care:** Prioritize self-care rituals that rejuvenate your mind and body, whether through leisure activities, hobbies, or relaxation techniques.
- **Healthy Boundaries:** Set boundaries to protect your time, energy, and emotional well-being from draining interactions.
- **Social Support:** Seek solace in the company of friends and family, fostering a network that provides emotional support.
- **Physical Activity:** Engage in regular exercise, which releases endorphins and acts as a natural stress-reliever.
- **Journaling:** Pouring your thoughts onto paper can provide catharsis and clarity, helping you process emotions and gain perspective.
- **Professional Support:** If stress and anxiety become overwhelming, consider seeking guidance from mental health professionals.

Practicing Mindfulness and Meditation

Mindfulness and meditation are ancient practices that offer modern-day tools for cultivating presence, emotional regulation, and mental clarity.

- **Mindfulness:** Mindfulness involves being fully present in the moment, observing thoughts, emotions, and sensations without judgment. Incorporate mindfulness into daily activities, like mindful eating or mindful walking.
- **Meditation:** Meditation is a dedicated practice that involves focusing your attention on a particular object, sound, or sensation. Regular meditation enhances emotional resilience, reduces anxiety, and fosters a sense of calm.
- **Breathing Exercises:** Deep breathing techniques, such as diaphragmatic breathing or the 4-7-8 technique, engage the body's relaxation response, promoting emotional balance.
- **Progressive** Muscle Relaxation: This practice involves tensing and then releasing muscle groups, promoting physical relaxation and emotional calmness.
- **Guided Imagery:** Visualization of peaceful scenes or positive outcomes can ease stress and elevate mood.
- **Loving-Kindness Meditation:** Also known as Metta meditation, this practice involves generating feelings of compassion and love toward oneself and others.

The Power of Emotional Intelligence

Emotional intelligence involves recognizing, understanding, and managing your emotions while empathizing with the emotions of others. Developing emotional intelligence enables you to navigate relationships with grace, make sound decisions, and foster a sense of contentment.

Creating Emotional Resilience

Emotional resilience is the ability to adapt and bounce back from adversity. It's cultivated through self-awareness, self-regulation, and a positive outlook. By developing emotional resilience, you fortify yourself against the storms of life, emerging stronger and wiser.

Conclusion: Cultivating Inner Equilibrium

In the tapestry of well-being, mental and emotional health are threads woven with intricate care. By nurturing your mind and emotions, you bolster your physical vitality and create a holistic foundation for a fulfilling life. The strategies explored in this chapter, from stress management to mindfulness and meditation, offer a compass to navigate the terrain of inner experiences. Through their transformative power, you cultivate a resilient spirit, an open heart, and a clear mind. As you journey towards mental and emotional equilibrium, you empower yourself to embrace life's complexities with a sense of grace and vitality that resonates through every facet of your being.

Chapter 9: Sustainable Lifestyle Changes:

- Making gradual and lasting changes
- Overcoming the challenges of maintaining new habits
- Creating a supportive environment for healthy living

Embarking on the path of healthy living is a journey of transformation, a testament to your commitment to nurturing your body, mind, and spirit. This chapter illuminates the art of making sustainable lifestyle changes, unravelling the threads of gradual transformation, overcoming challenges, and crafting an environment that nurtures your quest for well-being.

Making Gradual and Lasting Changes

Embrace Incremental Progress: The journey of a thousand miles begins with a single step. Embrace small, achievable changes rather than overwhelming overhauls. Gradual adjustments are more likely to become lasting habits.

- **Identify Priorities:** Reflect on your wellness goals and identify the most pressing areas for change. Prioritize these aspects and build upon them.

- **Set SMART Goals:** Specific, measurable, achievable, relevant, and time-bound (SMART) goals provide clarity and direction, helping you chart your progress.
- **Focus on Habits:** Shifting the focus from end results to daily habits fosters consistency. Habits form the foundation of sustained change.
- **Celebrate Small Wins:** Acknowledge and celebrate even minor achievements. These victories reinforce your motivation and commitment.
- **Practice Self-Compassion:** Be kind to yourself in the face of setbacks. Self-compassion fuels resilience and encourages you to continue your journey.

Overcoming the Challenges of Maintaining New Habits

- Mind the Motivation: Understand your reasons for change. Internal motivations rooted in personal values are more enduring than external pressures.
- Create Accountability: Share your goals with a friend, family member, or mentor who can provide encouragement and gentle accountability.
- Navigate Setbacks: Expect setbacks and view them as learning opportunities rather than failures. Analyse what led to the setback and adjust your approach.
- Address Obstacles: Identify obstacles that hinder your progress and develop strategies to overcome them. This proactive approach increases your resilience.
- Mind Over Matter: Cultivate a growth mindset, believing that your abilities and intelligence can be developed over time. This mindset encourages persistence.
- Refine and Adapt: As you progress, your needs and circumstances may change. Be willing to adapt your goals and strategies accordingly.

Creating a Supportive Environment for Healthy Living

- Surround Yourself with Positivity: Engage with individuals who uplift and support your journey. Limit interactions with those who undermine your efforts.
- Foster a Healthy Social Network: Cultivate relationships with like-minded individuals who share your wellness goals. Peer support can be invaluable.
- Incorporate Social Activities: Choose social activities that align with your healthy lifestyle, such as group fitness classes or healthy potlucks.
- Design a Nurturing Home Space: Create an environment that encourages your wellness journey. Keep healthy foods accessible and set up spaces for exercise and relaxation.
- Limit Temptations: Minimize exposure to unhealthy temptations, whether it's processed foods, excessive screen time, or negative influences.
- Seek Professional Guidance: Consult registered dietitians, fitness trainers, and mental health professionals for expert guidance tailored to your needs.

The Power of Habit Stacking

Habit stacking involves anchoring new habits to existing ones. By attaching new behaviours to familiar routines, you increase the likelihood of successful integration.

The Role of Mindfulness in Sustainable Change

Mindfulness offers a transformative lens through which to approach change. It encourages you to stay present, fully engage with your actions, and make intentional choices aligned with your values.

Cultivating Resilience Through Change

Resilience is the cornerstone of sustained change. It's the ability to bounce back from challenges, adapt to new circumstances, and stay committed to your goals.

Conclusion: An Ongoing Journey of Transformation

Sustainable lifestyle changes are a testament to your commitment to well-being, an acknowledgment of your inherent worthiness of a vibrant life. As you navigate the path of gradual transformation, surmount challenges, and cultivate a nurturing environment, you weave a tapestry of vitality that resonates through your physical, mental, and emotional dimensions. Remember, this journey is not a destination; it's an ongoing evolution, a sacred dance with change itself. In embracing this journey, you embrace yourself—unfolding, adapting, and growing with each step, each breath, each moment.

Chapter 10: Dining Out and Social Situations:

- Navigating healthy choices at restaurants
- Strategies for maintaining healthy habits during social events
- Balancing indulgence and moderation

Navigating the world of dining out and social gatherings can be a test of your commitment to healthy living. This chapter illuminates the art of making informed choices at restaurants, strategies for maintaining healthy habits during social events, and the delicate balance between indulgence and moderation.

Navigating Healthy Choices at Restaurants

Research Ahead: Review the restaurant's menu online to identify healthy options before arriving. Look for dishes with lean proteins, plenty of vegetables, and whole grains.

- **Control Portions:** Restaurants often serve larger portions than necessary. Consider sharing dishes with a friend or asking for a to-go container to portion out leftovers.
- **Customize Your Order:** Don't hesitate to customize your order. Ask for substitutions, such as replacing fries with a side salad or requesting grilled instead of fried options.

- **Be Mindful of Cooking Methods:** Opt for grilled, baked, steamed, or broiled dishes instead of fried or heavily sautéed options.
- **Limit Liquid Calories:** Be cautious with beverages; sugary sodas and alcoholic drinks can add unnecessary calories. Choose water, unsweetened tea, or sparkling water with a splash of citrus.
- **Watch Out for Hidden Ingredients:** Ask about ingredients or sauces that might not be listed on the menu. Some sauces can be high in sugars, sodium, and unhealthy fats.
- **Start with a Salad or Soup:** Begin your meal with a vegetable-based appetizer, like a salad or broth-based soup, to help control your appetite.
- **Practice Mindful Eating:** Eat slowly, savoring each bite. This helps you recognize when you're full, preventing overeating.

Strategies for Maintaining Healthy Habits During Social Events

Set Intentions: Decide in advance how you'll approach the event. Set a goal to make healthy choices while still enjoying the experience.

Eat Beforehand: Have a small, balanced meal or snack before attending an event. This can prevent overindulging due to hunger.

- **Survey the Options:** Take a look at all the food offerings before serving yourself. This allows you to choose the healthier options first.
- **Use Smaller Plates:** If available, choose a smaller plate for your food. This can help control portion sizes.
- **Engage in Conversation**: Engaging in conversations and socializing can slow down your eating pace, making it easier to recognize when you're full.
- **Stay Hydrated:** Drinking water throughout the event can help you feel full and prevent mindless snacking.
- **Practice the 80/20 Rule:** Strive to make healthy choices 80% of the time and allow yourself to indulge the remaining 20%.

Balancing Indulgence and Moderation

Practice Mindful Indulgence: If you choose to indulge, do so mindfully. Savor each bite and pay attention to how the food makes you feel.

- **Avoid Guilt:** Guilt can lead to a negative relationship with food. Enjoy your indulgence without judgment and move forward with your healthy habits.
- **Plan for Special Occasions: If** you know you'll be attending an event with indulgent foods, plan your meals earlier in the day to balance out your intake.
- **Focus on the Experience:** Instead of fixating solely on the food, focus on the overall experience of the event, including socializing and enjoying the ambiance.
- **Listen to Your Body:** Pay attention to your body's cues of hunger and fullness. Stop eating when you feel satisfied, not overly stuffed.
- **Practice Gratitude:** Approach indulgences with gratitude for the opportunity to enjoy special foods and experiences.

Creating a Balanced Approach

Finding the balance between enjoying social situations and maintaining healthy habits is an ongoing practice that requires mindfulness, self-awareness, and flexibility. By arming yourself with strategies to make informed choices, navigate social events, and indulge in moderation, you create a harmonious relationship with food and social occasions.

Conclusion: Savouring Every Bite and Moment

Dining out and social events are not just about what's on your plate; they're about relishing connections, savouring Flavors, and embracing the richness of life. By making conscious choices, practicing moderation, and prioritizing your overall well-being, you transform these occasions into opportunities for nourishment—of body, mind, and heart. In this chapter, you've uncovered the art of navigating these situations with grace, finding joy in every bite, and crafting a relationship with food that reflects your commitment to a vibrant and balanced life.

Chapter 11: Tracking Progress and Celebrating Success:

- The importance of tracking your health journey
- Setting milestones and celebrating achievements
- Adjusting your plan as needed for continuous improvement

The journey toward optimal health and well-being is a dynamic and transformative path. In this chapter, we explore the crucial role of tracking your health journey, setting meaningful milestones, and celebrating your achievements along the way. We'll also delve into the art of adjusting your plan as needed, ensuring continuous improvement and sustained progress.

The Importance of Tracking Your Health Journey

The Power of Awareness: Tracking your health journey offers a clear picture of where you started and where you're headed. It brings awareness to your habits, patterns, and progress.

- **Objective Feedback:** Data-driven tracking provides objective feedback, helping you make informed decisions based on tangible results rather than assumptions.
- **Motivation and Accountability:** Tracking fosters motivation as you witness your efforts translating into measurable improvements. It also enhances accountability by holding you responsible for your choices.
- **Identifying Trends and Patterns:** Regular tracking reveals trends and patterns, allowing you to identify what works well and areas that may require adjustment.
- **Evidence of Growth:** Looking back at your progress over time serves as a testament to your growth and commitment. It fuels your determination to continue the journey.

Setting Milestones and Celebrating Achievements

- Defining Meaningful Milestones: Establish short-term and long-term goals that reflect your aspirations. These milestones serve as guiding lights along your journey.

- SMART Goals Revisited: Create SMART goals—Specific, Measurable, Achievable, Relevant, and Time-bound. This framework ensures your milestones are clear and attainable.
- Focus on Non-Scale Victories: While weight-related goals are common, consider non-scale victories such as improved energy, increased strength, or better sleep.
- Celebrate Incremental Progress: Celebrate both small and large achievements. Each step forward, no matter how modest, is a testament to your commitment.
- Cultivating a Culture of Celebration: Embrace the practice of celebrating achievements with self-compassion and joy. These moments reinforce your motivation.

Adjusting Your Plan for Continuous Improvement

Evaluating Your Approach: Periodically assess your progress and the effectiveness of your strategies. Consider what's working well and what could be refined.

- Flexibility and Adaptability: Life is dynamic, and your health journey should reflect that. Be open to adjusting your plan based on changing circumstances.
- Reflect and Learn: Analyze setbacks and challenges as learning opportunities. Adjustments can help you overcome hurdles and grow stronger.
- Seeking Professional Guidance: If progress stalls or you encounter difficulties, consider seeking guidance from health professionals who can provide tailored advice.
- Intuitive Adjustments: As you become attuned to your body's signals and needs, you'll naturally refine your approach in alignment with your unique journey.

The Role of Mindfulness in Tracking and Celebrating

- Mindful Reflection: Regularly reflect on your journey with mindfulness. Observe your progress without judgment, acknowledging both successes and challenges.
- Cultivate Gratitude: Express gratitude for the progress you've made and the journey itself. Gratitude fuels positivity and amplifies your achievements.

- Present-Moment Awareness: Embrace the present moment as a culmination of your efforts. Celebrate where you are while remaining excited about the journey ahead.

A Holistic Approach to Progress and Success

Your health journey is not solely about physical changes; it encompasses your mental, emotional, and spiritual growth. As you track your progress, set milestones, and celebrate your achievements, remember that true success encompasses vitality, joy, and a balanced state of well-being.

Conclusion: Embracing Your Evolving Story

Tracking progress and celebrating success are integral parts of your health journey—a journey that unfolds as a tapestry of experiences, discoveries, and transformations. By mindfully observing your growth, setting meaningful milestones, and adapting your plan with flexibility, you honor the uniqueness of your path. This chapter encourages you to approach your journey as an ever-evolving story—one that's written with intention, woven with resilience, and adorned with the vibrant threads of progress and triumph. As you celebrate each step forward, you embody the essence of your journey—a celebration of health, vitality, and the unwavering commitment to becoming the best version of yourself.

Chapter 12: Long-Term Maintenance and Beyond:

- Strategies for sustaining healthy habits over time
- Dealing with setbacks and preventing relapses
- Embracing a lifelong commitment to well-being

As you journey through the chapters of healthy living, you come to the pinnacle of your quest: the realm of long-term maintenance and enduring well-being. This chapter delves into the art of sustaining healthy habits over time, addressing setbacks and preventing relapses, and embracing a lifelong commitment to your holistic well-being journey.

Here, you'll uncover the wisdom and strategies that empower you to navigate the ever-evolving landscape of your health.

Strategies for Sustaining Healthy Habits Over Time

Cultivate Consistency: Consistency is the cornerstone of long-term success. Commit to making healthy choices a natural part of your daily routine.

- **Embrace Variety**: Keep your journey vibrant by introducing new activities, foods, and practices. Variety prevents monotony and fosters ongoing engagement.
- **Set New Goals:** Continuously set new goals to maintain your motivation. Once you achieve a milestone, celebrate, and then define what's next on your path.
- **Reflect and Adjust:** Regularly reflect on your habits and progress. Adjust your strategies based on what's working well and areas that need refinement.
- **Practice Mindful Eating:** Continue practicing mindful eating, paying attention to hunger and fullness cues, even as your habits become second nature.
- **Prioritize Self-Care:** Nurture your emotional and mental well-being with self-care rituals that resonate with your evolving needs.

Dealing with Setbacks and Preventing Relapses

- **Shift Perspective on Setbacks:** View setbacks as opportunities for growth, not failures. Analyze the situation, learn from it, and use it as a stepping stone.
- **Mind Over Matter:** Adopt a growth mindset that acknowledges that setbacks are part of the journey. Your attitude influences your ability to bounce back.
- **Leverage Past Success**: Reflect on past successes to boost your confidence. Remind yourself that you've overcome challenges before and can do it again.
- **Seek Support:** Reach out to your support network when facing setbacks. Friends, family, or professionals can offer encouragement and perspective.

- **Identify Triggers:** Recognize triggers that lead to setbacks. Whether it's stress, emotions, or specific situations, being aware empowers you to navigate them.
- **Plan for Challenges:** Anticipate potential challenges and have strategies in place to overcome them. Preparedness is a key element of resilience.

Embracing a Lifelong Commitment to Well-being

A Dynamic Perspective: Embrace the notion that well-being is an ongoing journey. As circumstances change, your approach may also evolve.

- **Celebrate Your Evolution:** Recognize that your journey isn't static; it's a dynamic evolution. Celebrate how far you've come while embracing the path ahead.
- **Self-Compassion:** Practice self-compassion during every phase of your journey. Be gentle with yourself, whether you're facing challenges or enjoying success.
- **The Ebb and Flow:** Understand that well-being isn't linear. There will be periods of progress and plateaus. Embrace these cycles as part of the process.
- **Stay Connected to Your Why:** Regularly revisit your reasons for embarking on this journey. Your original motivations provide enduring guidance and purpose.
- **Continual Learning:** Approach your journey as an ongoing learning experience. Stay curious and open to discovering new strategies and insights.

The Role of Mindfulness in Long-Term Maintenance

- **Mindful Self-Reflection:** Periodically reflect on your journey with mindfulness. Observe your progress, setbacks, and growth without judgment.
- **Present-Moment Awareness:** Anchor yourself in the present, appreciating the beauty of each moment while acknowledging the journey's continual flow.
- **Mindful Adaptation:** Use mindfulness to adapt your strategies as needed. Tune into your body's signals and respond with intuitive adjustments.

The Symphony of a Lifelong Journey

Embracing long-term maintenance is akin to conducting a symphony. You are both the composer and the conductor, orchestrating the harmonious balance of health and well-being. Just as a symphony evolves through intricate melodies and harmonies, your journey evolves through varied experiences, emotions, and choices.

Conclusion: The Legacy of Enduring Well-being

As you delve into the realm of long-term maintenance, you create a legacy—a testament to your commitment, resilience, and capacity for growth. Your journey transcends the boundaries of time, encompassing the past, present, and future. Through strategies, setbacks, and successes, you weave a tapestry of enduring well-being—an expression of your ongoing dedication to a life that thrives on all levels. By nurturing your body, mind, and spirit, you not only embrace a vibrant existence but also inspire others to embark on their own transformative journeys. This chapter concludes your expedition through the landscape of holistic health—a journey that now extends into the boundless horizon of possibilities that lie beyond.

Conclusion:

- Reflecting on your journey to healthy living
- The ongoing benefits of maintaining healthy habits
- Encouragement to continue evolving and thriving

As you come to the end of this guide—a compass through the labyrinth of healthy living—you find yourself at a crossroads. The culmination of your journey is not an endpoint but a pause—a moment of reflection, gratitude, and anticipation for the limitless possibilities that lie ahead. This conclusion invites you to gaze back at the footprints you've left on the sands of well-being, to recognize the ongoing benefits of maintaining your healthy habits, and to step forward with the conviction to continue evolving and thriving.

Reflecting on Your Journey to Healthy Living

Pause for a moment and reflect on the path you've traversed. Remember the determination that fueled your first step and the curiosity that guided you through each chapter. Recall the challenges you conquered, the discoveries you made, and the transformations you embraced. Every choice, every decision, and every effort has woven together to create the tapestry of your personal well-being journey. You've embarked on a pilgrimage that extends beyond physical changes— it's an odyssey of growth, resilience, and self-discovery.

The Ongoing Benefits of Maintaining Healthy Habits

As you carry the torch of your health journey into the future, recognize the ongoing benefits that accompany your commitment to maintaining healthy habits.

- **Physical Vitality**: Your body is a vessel that carries you through life's adventures. By nourishing it with wholesome foods and regular exercise, you foster energy, strength, and longevity.
- **Mental Clarity:** A healthy lifestyle nurtures your mind, enhancing cognitive function, focus, and emotional resilience. Clarity of thought becomes your compass in navigating life's complexities.
- **Emotional Equilibrium:** Your journey has also been one of nurturing emotional well-being. Through mindfulness, self-care, and self-compassion, you've cultivated a balanced emotional landscape.
- **Spiritual Wholeness:** Your well-being journey encompasses your spirit as well. As you prioritize self-care, you tap into your inner wellspring of peace, joy, and connection.
- **Positive Influence:** Your journey ripples outward, inspiring others to embrace their own paths to well-being. By embodying health, you become a beacon of possibility for those around you.

Encouragement to Continue Evolving and Thriving

As you step beyond this guide, remember that your journey doesn't end—it evolves. Embrace the ever-blooming potential that resides within you:

- **Celebrate Every Moment**: Embrace the present moment as a canvas for mindful living. Celebrate each choice you make, for they shape your path.
- **Embrace the Process:** Your journey is not linear; it's a symphony of growth. Embrace setbacks as stepping stones and plateaus as opportunities for reflection.
- **Prioritize Self-Care:** Nurture your well-being through self-care rituals that nourish your body, mind, and soul. Prioritize your needs without guilt.
- **Stay Curious:** Approach your journey with an insatiable curiosity. Continually seek new knowledge, explore new activities, and evolve your habits.
- **Seek Connection:** Engage with a supportive community of like-minded individuals. Connection fuels your commitment and reminds you that you're not alone.
- **Practice Self-Compassion:** Be kind to yourself as you navigate life's challenges. Self-compassion is the elixir that sustains your resilience.
- **Create Your Unique Path:** Your journey is as unique as your fingerprint. Be open to adapting your approach based on your individual needs and circumstances.

The Ever-Evolving Symphony of Your Life

As you step forward, remember that your journey is a symphony—an intricate composition of moments, choices, and experiences. Just as a symphony evolves through crescendos and diminuendos, your journey weaves through peaks and valleys. You are the conductor, embracing the ebb and flow with grace and resilience.

Embrace the Legacy You're Creating

Every choice you make, every habit you cultivate, and every moment of mindfulness you practice weaves the legacy of your well-being. You're authoring a story of vitality, balance, and growth—a legacy that extends far beyond your individual journey.

A Final Word of Gratitude

Thank you for embarking on this journey—a journey that's not just about health but about becoming the best version of yourself. Your commitment to your well-being radiates a ripple effect that touches lives beyond measure. May you continue to flourish, evolve, and thrive, embracing the richness of each day, and nurturing the symphony of your ever-blossoming well-being.

Appendix: Empowering Your Well-being Journey

- Sample meal plans and recipes
- Resources for further reading and exploration
- Worksheets and tools to aid in goal setting and tracking

Welcome to the appendix—a treasure trove of resources designed to empower your well-being journey beyond the pages of this guide. Here, you'll find sample meal plans and recipes to inspire your culinary adventures, a curated list of resources for further reading and exploration, and a collection of worksheets and tools to aid in goal setting and tracking. Consider this your toolkit for continuous growth, self-discovery, and vibrant living.

Sample Meal Plans and Recipes

Balanced Breakfasts:

- Overnight oats with berries and nuts
- Scrambled eggs with spinach and whole-grain toast
- Greek yogurt parfait with fruit and granola

Lunches On-the-Go:

- Quinoa salad with mixed vegetables and a protein source
- Veggie wrap with hummus, avocado, and greens
- Lentil soup with a side of whole-grain crackers

Dinner Delights:

- Grilled chicken or tofu with roasted vegetables and quinoa
- Baked salmon with steamed broccoli and sweet potatoes
- Stir-fried vegetables with lean beef and brown rice

Snacks to Fuel Your Day:

- Apple slices with almond butter
- Greek yogurt with honey and walnuts
- Hummus with carrot and cucumber sticks

Resources for Further Reading and Exploration

Books:

- "The Blue Zones Solution" by Dan Buettner
- "Atomic Habits" by James Clear
- "Mindful Eating" by Jan Chozen Bays

Websites and Blogs:

- Harvard Health Blog (health.harvard.edu/blog)
- Nutrition Stripped (nutritionstripped.com)
- Mindful.org (mindful.org)

Podcasts:

- The Nutrition Diva's Quick and Dirty Tips for Eating Well and Feeling Fabulous
- The Minimalists (theminimalists.com/podcast)

Worksheets and Tools for Goal Setting and Tracking

Goal-Setting Worksheet: A guided worksheet to help you set specific, measurable, achievable, relevant, and time-bound (SMART) goals for your well-being journey.

Habit Tracker: A tool to monitor the consistency of your daily habits and track your progress over time.

Meal Planning Template: An organized template to plan your meals and snacks for the week, ensuring balanced nutrition.

Mindful Eating Journal: A journal to record your experiences and reflections as you practice mindful eating.

Self-Care Planner: A planner to schedule and prioritize self-care activities that nurture your emotional and mental well-being.

Conclusion: Empowerment at Your Fingertips

As you peruse the resources within this appendix, remember that empowerment lies at your fingertips. Whether you're experimenting with new recipes, diving into insightful books, exploring informative websites, or utilizing tools for goal setting and tracking, you're taking ownership of your journey. This appendix invites you to forge your unique path, tapping into your inner wellspring of curiosity, determination, and growth. May these resources be your companions, guiding lights, and allies as you continue to evolve, thrive, and embrace the vibrant symphony of your well-being.

Congratulations for your happy & healthy life…..

www.ingramcontent.com/pod-product-compliance
Lightning Source LLC
Chambersburg PA
CBHW060901260726
48661CB00008B/3383